MENOPAUSE DIET PLAN COOK BOOK

Essential Tips and Delicious Recipes for the Menopause Diet Plan Cook Book

REX LEWIS

Table of Contents

Introduction

Menopause Is An Inherent Physiological Process That Signifies The Conclusion Of A Woman's Menstrual Periods And Ability To Conceive. It Generally Manifests In The Late 40s Or Early 50s. Menopause Is Characterized By Hormonal Fluctuations, Specifically A Decrease In Estrogen Levels, Which Can Result In A Range Of Symptoms Including Hot Flashes, Mood Swings, Sleep Disruptions, And Alterations In Metabolism. An Optimal And Well-Rounded Diet Can Have A Pivotal Impact On Treating These Symptoms And Promoting General Well-Being Throughout This Transitional Phase.

Below Are Few Dietary Factors To Consider During Menopause:

• **Calcium And Vitamin D:** Women May Undergo A Decline In Bone Density After Menopause As A Result Of Hormonal Changes. It Is Crucial To Consume Foods That Are High In Calcium And Vitamin D In Order To Maintain Good Bone Health. Excellent Sources Of Essential Nutrients Include Dairy Products, Such As Milk And Cheese, Leafy Green Vegetables, Fortified Plant-Based Milk, And Fatty Fish.

• **Whole Grains:** Whole Grains Are An Excellent Source Of Dietary Fiber And Can Aid In Weight Management, Lower The Likelihood Of Heart

Disease, And Maintain Stable Blood Sugar Levels. Some Examples Of Nutritious Grains Are Brown Rice, Quinoa, Whole Wheat, Oats, And Barley.

• Incorporate Lean Protein Sources Into Your Diet, Such As Poultry, Fish, Tofu, Lentils, And Nuts. Protein Has A Crucial Role In Preserving Muscle Mass, Boosting Metabolism, And Creating A Sensation Of Satiety.

• Consuming A Diet Abundant In Fruits And Vegetables Offers Vital Vitamins, Minerals, And Antioxidants. These Substances Can Mitigate Oxidative Stress And Promote Overall Well-Being. Strive To Consume A Range Of Vibrant Fruits And Vegetables In

Order To Guarantee A Diverse Intake Of Essential Nutrients.

• Incorporate Sources Of Nutritious Fats Into Your Diet, Such As Avocados, Nuts, Seeds, And Olive Oil. Omega-3 Fatty Acids, Included In Fatty Fish Such As Salmon, Can Promote Cardiovascular Well-Being And Decrease Inflammation.

• **Hydration:** Ensure Optimal Hydration By Consuming Ample Amounts Of Water. Proper Hydration Is Crucial For Maintaining Good Health And Can Also Provide Relief From Symptoms Such As Hot Flashes And Dry Skin.

• Restrict The Intake Of Caffeine And Alcohol: O Consuming Excessive Amounts Of Coffee And Alcohol Can Worsen Symptoms Such As Hot Flashes And Disturb Sleep. Restricting Consumption May Aid In The Management Of These Symptoms.

• Weight Management;. Sustaining A Healthy Weight Might Mitigate Certain Symptoms Associated With Menopause, Such As Joint Discomfort And Sleep Disruptions. Weight Management Requires Adhering To A Balanced Diet And Engaging In Regular Physical Activity.

• It Is Advisable To Restrict The Consumption Of Processed Foods And Added Sugars Due To Their Potential

To Cause Weight Gain And Have Adverse Effects On General Well-Being.

• Seek Guidance From A Healthcare Professional: Individual Dietary Requirements Can Differ, And It Is Recommended To Seek Assistance From A Healthcare Professional Or A Certified Dietitian For Individualized Recommendations Based On Your Health Condition And Specific Needs During Menopause.

Aside From Nutritional Factors, Consistent Physical Activity, Effective Stress Control, And Adequate Sleep Also Contribute Significantly To Promoting General Well-Being Throughout The Menopausal Period. It

Is Crucial To View Menopause As A
Distinct Stage In A Woman's Life, And
A Comprehensive Approach To Health
Is Important.

CHAPTER ONE
Definition and Phases

Menopause Is The Cessation Of A Woman's Reproductive Capacity, Signifying The Conclusion Of Her Fertile Years. Menopause Is The State Of Permanent End Of Menstruation And Fertility, Usually Happening In The Late 40s Or Early 50s. Menopause Is Marked By Hormonal Changes, Notably A Decrease In The Synthesis Of Estrogen And Progesterone By The Ovaries.

Stages Of Menopause: Menopause Is Characterized By A Steady Progression Through Several Phases, Rather Than Occurring Suddenly. These Stages Are

Commonly Classified In The Following Manner:

• Perimenopause Refers To The Transitional Phase Leading Up To Menopause: This Stage Commences Several Years Before To Menopause. It Is Characterized By Erratic Menstrual Periods And Varying Hormone Levels. During Perimenopause, Women May Encounter Symptoms Such As Hot Flashes, Nocturnal Sweats, Mood Swings, And Alterations In Libido. The Onset Of This Condition Typically Occurs In The Late 30s Or Early 40s And Last Till Menopause.

• **Menopause:** Menopause Is Defined As The State In Which A Woman Has Not Experienced A Menstrual Period

For A Continuous Duration Of 12 Months. The Mean Age Of Spontaneous Menopause Is Approximately 51, However There Can Be Significant Variation. At This Stage, The Ovaries Stop Releasing Eggs, And The Levels Of Estrogen And Progesterone Stay Persistently Low.

• Postmenopause Is The Term Used To Describe The Phase That Comes After Menopause. During This Stage, The Symptoms Of Menopause May Persist Or Decrease, And The Woman Adapts To The Hormonal Fluctuations. Postmenopausal Women May Have An Elevated Chance Of Developing Certain Health Conditions, Such As Osteoporosis And Cardiovascular

Disease. It Encompasses The Remaining Duration Of A Woman's Life.

It Is Crucial To Acknowledge That The Individual Experiences Of Menopause Can Differ. Certain Women May Undergo This Shift With Negligible Symptoms, But Others May Encounter More Conspicuous Alterations. In Addition, Menopause May Occur Prematurely As A Result Of Factors Such As Genetic Predisposition, Surgical Interventions (E.G., Hysterectomy), Or Medical Therapies Such As Chemotherapy. Women Should Seek Guidance From Healthcare Professionals To Effectively Address Symptoms And

Uphold Their General Well-Being During This Particular Phase Of Life.

Hormonal Changes

Hormonal Changes Are A Central Aspect Of The Menopausal Transition. The Primary Hormones Affected During Menopause Are Estrogen And Progesterone, Which Are Produced By The Ovaries. These Hormonal Shifts Can Lead To Various Physical And Physiological Changes. Here's An Overview Of The Hormonal Changes That Occur During Menopause:

Estrogen Decline:

• Estrogen, A Key Female Sex Hormone, Plays A Crucial Role In Regulating The Menstrual Cycle,

Supporting Reproductive Health, And Influencing Various Bodily Functions. During Perimenopause And Menopause, The Ovaries Gradually Produce Less Estrogen. This Decline Can Lead To Irregular Menstrual Cycles And Eventually Result In The Cessation Of Menstruation.

Progesterone Decline:

• Progesterone Is Another Hormone Produced By The Ovaries, And Its Levels Also Decline During Menopause. Progesterone Is Involved In Preparing The Uterine Lining For Pregnancy. As Hormonal Balance Shifts, Decreased Progesterone Contributes To Changes In The Menstrual Cycle.

Follicle-Stimulating Hormone (FSH) Increase:

As Estrogen Levels Decrease, The Pituitary Gland Releases More Follicle-Stimulating Hormone (FSH) To Stimulate The Ovaries To Produce Estrogen. Elevated FSH Levels Are A Characteristic Marker Of Menopause And Can Be Measured Through Blood Tests.

Luteinizing Hormone (LH) Increase:

• Similar To FSH, Luteinizing Hormone (LH) Levels May Increase During Menopause. LH Plays A Role In Regulating The Menstrual Cycle And Is Involved In Ovulation.

Androgen Levels:

• While Estrogen And Progesterone Levels Decline Significantly, The Production Of Androgens (Male Sex Hormones Like Testosterone) May Relatively Decrease But Not Cease Entirely. This Can Influence Libido And Other Aspects Of Sexual Health.

• These Hormonal Changes Contribute To The Various Symptoms Experienced During Menopause, Including:

• **Hot Flashes And Night Sweats:** Fluctuating Hormone Levels Can Disrupt The Body's Temperature Regulation, Leading To Sudden Sensations Of Heat And Sweating.

• **Vaginal Dryness:** Declining Estrogen Levels Can Result In A Decrease In Vaginal Lubrication, Leading To Discomfort And Potential Issues With Sexual Activity.

• **Mood Swings And Sleep Disturbances:** Hormonal Fluctuations Can Impact Neurotransmitters In The Brain, Contributing To Mood Swings, Irritability, And Sleep Disturbances.

• **Changes In Bone Density:** Estrogen Plays A Role In Maintaining Bone Density, So Its Decline Can Contribute To An Increased Risk Of Osteoporosis.

• **Changes In Skin And Hair:** Hormonal Changes Can Affect The Skin's Elasticity And Moisture, Leading

To Changes In Skin Texture. Hair May Also Become Thinner.

Management Of Menopausal Symptoms Often Involves Addressing Hormonal Changes Through Hormone Replacement Therapy (HRT) Or Other Medications. Lifestyle Modifications, Including A Healthy Diet, Regular Exercise, And Stress Management, Can Also Help Alleviate Symptoms And Support Overall Well-Being During This Transition. Consulting With Healthcare Professionals Is Crucial For Personalized Guidance And Treatment Options Based On Individual Health Needs And Preferences.

Common Symptoms

Menopause Is Characterized By A Range Of Symptoms, And The Intensity And Length Of These Symptoms Can Differ Significantly Across Individuals. The Prevailing Symptoms Encompass:

1. Irregular Menstrual Cycles: During the Perimenopausal Stage, Women May Experience Irregular Menstrual Cycles Characterized By Fluctuations In The Length And Intensity Of Their Periods. This Is Frequently One Of The Initial Indications Of The Onset Of Menopause.

2. Hot Flashes And Night Sweats, Characterized By Abrupt And Intense Sensations Of Heat, Frequently

Accompanied By Perspiration, Are Prevalent Symptoms Experienced During Menopause. Nocturnal Vasomotor Symptoms, Commonly Known As Night Sweats, Can Cause Sleep Disruptions Due To Episodes Of Sudden And Intense Heat Sensations, Also Known As Hot Flashes, That Can Occur Either During The Day Or At Night.

3. Vaginal Dryness And Pain: Decreased Levels Of Estrogen Can Cause Alterations In The Vaginal Tissue, Resulting In Dryness, Itching, And Pain. This Might Lead To Discomfort During Sexual Intercourse.

4. Sleep Disturbances: Hormonal Fluctuations, Nocturnal Perspiration,

And Various Other Factors Can Interfere With Sleep Cycles, Resulting In Challenges With Both Initiating And Maintaining Sleep.

5. Mood Swings And Irritation Can Occur Due To The Fluctuation Of Hormone Levels, Which Can Impact The Neurotransmitters In The Brain And Result In Changes In Emotional Well-Being.

6. Exhaustion: Hormonal Fluctuations, Disruptions In Sleep Patterns, And Various Other Variables Can Contribute To Sensations Of Exhaustion And Diminished Energy Levels.

7. Difficulty Concentrating: Some Women May Encounter Challenges With Memory And Focus After Menopause, Commonly Known As "Menopausal Cognitive Impairment."

8. Joint Pain And Muscle Aches: Hormonal Fluctuations During Menopause Can Potentially Lead To The Occurrence Of Joint Pain And Muscle Aches.

9. Alterations in Libido: Variations In Hormone Levels, Specifically Estrogen And Androgens, Can Influence Sexual Desire And Contentment.

10. Urine Changes: Alterations In The Anatomy And Physiology Of The Urine System Might Result In Symptoms

Such As Heightened Frequency Of Urination And Urinary Incontinence.

11. Weight Gain: Metabolic Alterations And Hormonal Oscillations Can Contribute To Alterations In Body Composition And An Increase In Weight, Especially In The Abdomen Region.

12. Skin And Hair Alterations: Reduced Collagen Synthesis And Fluctuations In Hormone Levels Can Impact The Flexibility And Hydration Of The Skin, Resulting In Modifications To Its Texture. Hair May Experience A Reduction In Thickness.

It Is Noteworthy That Not Every Woman Will Encounter All Of These

Symptoms, And The Severity Of These Symptoms Can Differ. In Addition, The Duration Of Symptoms Might Vary, With Certain Women Experiencing Them For A Relatively Brief Period, While Others May Have Symptoms That Endure For Several Years. Implementing Lifestyle Improvements, Such As Adopting A Nutritious Diet, Engaging In Consistent Physical Activity, Effectively Managing Stress, And Ensuring Sufficient Sleep, Can Assist In Effectively Managing Certain Symptoms. In Cases With More Severe Symptoms, Medical Measures Such As Hormone Replacement Therapy (HRT) Or Other Drugs May Be Advised. Seeking Advice From Healthcare Specialists Is Essential For Obtaining

Specialized Counsel And Treatment Alternatives Tailored To One's Specific Health Requirements And Preferences.

CHAPTER TWO
Importance of Nutrition during Menopause

Proper Nutrition Is Essential During Menopause To Promote Overall Well-Being, Alleviate Symptoms, And Lower The Likelihood Of Specific Health Concerns. During Menopause, It Is Crucial For Women To Be Mindful Of Their Food Choices Due To The Hormonal Changes They Experience. Here Are Several Crucial Factors Emphasizing The Significance Of Nutrition During Menopause:

1. Bone Health: The Reduction In Estrogen Levels During Menopause Is Linked To A Deterioration In Bone Density, Resulting In An Elevated

Susceptibility To Osteoporosis And Fractures. Sufficient Consumption Of Calcium And Vitamin D Is Essential For Preserving Bone Health. These Important Elements Can Be Obtained From Dairy Products, Leafy Green Vegetables, Fortified Foods, And Supplements.

2. Heart Health: Menopausal Hormonal Fluctuations Can Impact Cardiovascular Well-Being. Consuming A Diet That Is Beneficial For Heart Health, Consisting Of An Abundance Of Fruits, Vegetables, Whole Grains, And Lean Proteins, Can Effectively Regulate Cholesterol Levels And Decrease The Likelihood Of Developing Heart Disease. Omega-3 Fatty Acids Derived

From Fatty Fish, Flaxseeds, And Walnuts Can Also Promote Cardiovascular Well-Being.

3. Weight Management: Hormonal Fluctuations During Menopause Can Lead To An Increase In Body Weight, Especially In The Abdomen Region. Incorporating A Diverse Range Of Nutrient-Rich Foods Into One's Diet, Combined With Consistent Physical Activity, Can Effectively Control Weight And Promote Overall Health And Wellness.

4. Blood Sugar Regulation: The Likelihood Of Developing Insulin Resistance And Type 2 Diabetes May Be Higher During And After Menopause. Opting For Complex

Carbs, Meals Abundant In Fiber, And Sustaining A Desirable Weight Can Aid In The Regulation Of Blood Sugar Levels.

5. Management Of Hot Flashes: Certain Foods And Beverages, Including As Spicy Meals, Caffeine, And Alcohol, Might Act As Triggers Or Worsen Hot Flashes. Regulating The Consumption Of These Things And Choosing A Diet That Is Balanced In Nutrients Can Aid In Decreasing The Occurrence And Severity Of Hot Flashes.

6. Hormonal Balance: Certain Nutrients, Such Phytoestrogens Included In Soy Products, Provide A Slight Estrogenic Impact And Can

Assist In Relieving Specific Symptoms Associated With Menopause. Adding Diverse Range Of Plant-Based Foods Containing These Chemicals Can Help Maintain Hormonal Equilibrium.

7. Maintaining Vaginal And Urinary Health Can Be Supported By Ensuring Proper Hydration And Consuming A Diet That Includes Foods With High Water Content. In Addition, The Consumption Of Probiotic-Rich Foods, Such As Yogurt And Fermented Foods Can Potentially Enhance The Health Of The Vaginal Microbiota.

8. Mood And Cognitive Performance: Consuming Meals That Are Rich In Nutrients, Particularly Those That Contain High Levels Of

Antioxidants And Omega-3 Fatty Acids, Can Potentially Enhance Mood And Cognitive Performance. Incorporating A Diverse Range Of Vibrant Fruits, Vegetables, And Oily Fish Into One's Diet Can Supply Crucial Nutrients That Support Brain Function.

9. Gut Health: Menopausal Hormonal Fluctuations Can Impact The State Of The Gastrointestinal System. Incorporating Foods That Are High In Fiber And Include Probiotics Into One's Diet Can Promote A Healthy Gut Microbiota, Which Is Crucial For Proper Digestion And Overall Health.

10. Overall Well-Being: Optimal Overall Well-Being Is Contingent Upon

Maintaining A Well-Balanced And Healthy Diet. It Supplies The Body With Essential Nutrients To Sustain Energy Levels, Enhance Immunological Function, And Optimize Organ Function.

Women Experiencing Menopause Should Seek Advice From Healthcare Professionals Or Trained Dietitians To Receive Tailored Guidance That Takes Into Account Their Specific Health Requirements And Preferences. Engaging In Well-Informed Dietary Decision-Making And Embracing A Healthy Lifestyle Can Have A Beneficial Effect On The Menopausal Journey And Promote Long-Term Well-Being.

Key Nutrients for Menopausal Women

During Menopause, Maintaining A Well-Balanced And Nutrient-Dense Diet Is Crucial For Supporting Overall Health And Managing Specific Symptoms Associated With This Life Stage. Here Are Key Nutrients That Are Particularly Important For Menopausal Women:

• **Calcium:** Adequate Calcium Intake Is Essential For Maintaining Bone Health, Especially As Estrogen Levels Decline During Menopause. Good Sources Of Calcium Include Dairy Products, Fortified Plant-Based Milk, Leafy Green Vegetables, And Fortified Foods.

- **Vitamin D:** Vitamin D Works In Conjunction With Calcium To Support Bone Health. It Helps The Body Absorb Calcium And Promotes Bone Mineralization. Exposure To Sunlight Is A Natural Source Of Vitamin D, And Dietary Sources Include Fatty Fish, Fortified Dairy Or Plant-Based Milk, And Vitamin D Supplements.

- **Magnesium:** Magnesium Is Important For Bone Health, Muscle Function, And Energy Metabolism. Good Dietary Sources Of Magnesium Include Nuts, Seeds, Whole Grains, Leafy Green Vegetables, And Legumes.

- **Omega-3 Fatty Acids:** Omega-3 Fatty Acids Have Anti-Inflammatory Properties And Can Support Heart Health. Fatty Fish Such As Salmon, Mackerel, And Sardines, As Well As Flaxseeds, Chia Seeds, And Walnuts, Are Good Sources Of Omega-3s.

- **Phytoestrogens:** Phytoestrogens Are Plant Compounds That Have Mild Estrogenic Effects And May Help Alleviate Certain Menopausal Symptoms. Foods Rich In Phytoestrogens Include Soy Products (Tofu, Soy Milk), Flaxseeds, Whole Grains, And Legumes.

- **Vitamin K:** Vitamin K Is Important For Bone Health And Plays A Role In Blood Clotting. Green Leafy Vegetables, Such As Kale, Spinach, And Broccoli, Are Good Sources Of Vitamin K.

- **Vitamin C:** Vitamin C Is An Antioxidant That Supports The Immune System And Helps The Body Absorb Iron From Plant-Based Foods. Citrus Fruits, Strawberries, Bell Peppers, And Broccoli Are Excellent Sources Of Vitamin C.

- **B Vitamins:** B Vitamins, Including B6, B12, And Folate, Play A Role In Energy Metabolism And Support Nervous System Function. Whole Grains, Lean Meats, Fish, Poultry,

Dairy Products, And Leafy Green Vegetables Are Good Sources Of B Vitamins.

• **Iron:** Iron Is Important For Transporting Oxygen In The Blood. While The Need For Iron Decreases After Menopause Due To The Cessation Of Menstrual Bleeding, It's Still Important To Include Iron-Rich Foods Like Lean Meats, Legumes, And Fortified Cereals In The Diet.

• **Protein:** Adequate Protein Intake Is Crucial For Maintaining Muscle Mass, Supporting Metabolism, And Promoting Overall Health. Include Sources Of Lean Protein Such As Poultry, Fish, Tofu, Legumes, And Nuts In Your Diet.

- **Fiber:** Fiber Helps Maintain Digestive Health And Regulate Blood Sugar Levels. Whole Grains, Fruits, Vegetables, Legumes, And Nuts Are Excellent Sources Of Dietary Fiber.

- **Water:** Staying Well-Hydrated Is Important For Overall Health, Especially As Hormonal Changes During Menopause Can Impact Skin And Urinary Health.

Menopausal Women Should Prioritize Incorporating A Diverse And Balanced Diet That Encompasses A Wide Array Of Nutrient-Dense Foods. Furthermore, Seeking Advice From Healthcare Specialists Or Qualified Dietitians Can Offer Tailored Recommendations That Take Into

Account Specific Health Requirements
And Personal Preferences Throughout
Menopause.

CHAPTER THREE
Creating a Well-Balanced Meal Plan

To Develop A Well-Rounded Meal Plan For Menopausal Women, It Is Important To Include A Diverse Range Of Foods That Are High In Nutrients. This Will Help To Promote General Health And Effectively Manage The Symptoms That Are Commonly Experienced During This Period Of Life. Below Is An Exemplar Eating Plan For A Day, Emphasizing Essential Nutrients And Dietary Considerations Specifically For Menopause:

Breakfast:

Whole Grain Oatmeal:

- Cooked With Water Or Milk (Dairy Or Fortified Plant-Based Milk)
- Topped With Sliced Bananas Or Berries For Added Fiber And Vitamins
- Sprinkle Ground Flaxseeds Or Chia Seeds For Omega-3 Fatty Acids

Greek Yogurt:

- Provides Calcium And Probiotics For Gut Health
- Add A Handful Of Almonds Or Walnuts For Added Protein And Healthy Fats

Green Tea:

- A Low-Calorie Beverage Rich In Antioxidants, May Help With Weight Management And Reduce Hot Flashes

Mid-Morning Snack:

Apple Slices with Almond Butter:

- Provides Fiber, Vitamins, And Minerals From The Apple
- Almond Butter Adds Protein And Healthy Fats For Satiety

Lunch:

Grilled Chicken Salad:

- Mixed Greens (Spinach, Arugula, Kale) For Fiber and Vitamins

- Grilled Chicken Breast For Lean Protein

- Sliced Avocado For Healthy Fats And Potassium

- Cherry Tomatoes, Cucumbers, And Bell Peppers For Added Nutrients

Quinoa or Whole Grain Bread:

- Served On The Side To Provide Complex Carbohydrates And Additional Fiber

Afternoon Snack:

Vegetable Sticks with Hummus:

- Carrot, Cucumber, And Bell Pepper Sticks For Crunch And Fiber

- Hummus Provides Protein And Healthy Fats

Dinner:

Salmon Fillet:

- Rich In Omega-3 Fatty Acids For Heart And Bone Health
- Baked Or Grilled With Herbs And Lemon

Roasted Vegetables:

- Mix Of Colorful Vegetables Such As Broccoli, Cauliflower, Carrots, And Brussels Sprouts
- Drizzle With Olive Oil And Season With Herbs And Spices

Quinoa or Brown Rice:

- Served As a Side Dish To Provide Complex Carbohydrates And Additional Fiber

Evening Snack:

Yogurt Parfait:

- Greek Yogurt Layered With Mixed Berries And A Sprinkle Of Granola
- Provides Calcium, Probiotics, Fiber, And Antioxidants

Hydration:

Water: Drink Plenty Of Water Throughout The Day To Stay Hydrated

Herbal Teas: Enjoy Herbal Teas Such As Chamomile Or Peppermint For Relaxation And Hydration

Additional Considerations:

• Aim To Include A Variety Of Colorful Fruits And Vegetables Throughout The Day To Ensure A Diverse Intake Of Vitamins, Minerals, And Antioxidants.

• Choose Lean Protein Sources Such As Poultry, Fish, Tofu, Legumes, And Nuts To Support Muscle Health And Metabolism.

• Incorporate Whole Grains Such As Oats, Quinoa, Brown Rice, And Whole Grain Bread To Provide Complex Carbohydrates, Fiber, And Essential Nutrients.

• Limit Processed Foods, Added Sugars, And Excessive Salt Intake To Support Overall Health And Manage Symptoms Such As Weight Gain And Bloating.

• Consider Incorporating Foods Rich In Phytoestrogens Such As Soy Products, Flaxseeds, And Legumes To Support Hormonal Balance.

This Meal Plan Offers A Well-Balanced Combination Of Macronutrients (Carbohydrates, Proteins, And Fats) And Micronutrients (Vitamins And Minerals) To Promote General Health And Well-Being Throughout Menopause. Modify Serving Sizes And Meal Selections According To Personal Preferences, Nutritional

Requirements, And Levels Of Physical Activity. Seeking Advice From A Healthcare Practitioner Or Qualified Dietitian Can Offer Individualized Direction And Assistance In Controlling Menopausal Symptoms Through Dietary Choices.

Recommended Foods

Adopting A Nutritious And Well-Balanced Diet During Menopause Entails Including Foods That Are High In Nutrients To Promote Overall Health And Assist In Managing Specific Symptoms Related To This Phase Of Life. Here Are Some Foods That Are Beneficial To Consume During Menopause:

Fruits and Vegetables:

• Colorful Fruits And Vegetables Provide Essential Vitamins, Minerals, Antioxidants, And Fiber. Aim For A Variety Of Options To Ensure A Diverse Nutrient Intake.

Leafy Greens:

• Dark Leafy Greens Like Spinach, Kale, And Swiss Chard Are Rich In Calcium, Magnesium, And Vitamin K, Supporting Bone Health.

Whole Grains:

• Whole Grains Like Quinoa, Brown Rice, Oats, And Whole Wheat Provide Complex Carbohydrates, Fiber, And Various Nutrients. They Contribute To

Sustained Energy Levels And Digestive Health.

Fatty Fish:

• Fatty Fish Such As Salmon, Mackerel, And Sardines Are Excellent Sources Of Omega-3 Fatty Acids. These Fatty Acids Support Heart Health, Reduce Inflammation, And May Help Manage Mood Swings.

Lean Proteins:

• Incorporate Lean Protein Sources Like Poultry, Fish, Tofu, Legumes, And Nuts. Protein Is Essential For Maintaining Muscle Mass, Supporting Metabolism, And Providing A Feeling Of Fullness.

Dairy or Fortified Plant-Based Milk:

• Calcium And Vitamin D Are Crucial For Bone Health. Include Dairy Products Or Fortified Plant-Based Milk To Ensure An Adequate Intake Of These Nutrients.

Soy Products:

• Foods Like Tofu, Edamame, And Soy Milk Contain Phytoestrogens, Which May Help Alleviate Certain Menopausal Symptoms Due To Their Mild Estrogenic Effects.

Nuts and Seeds:

• Almonds, Walnuts, Flaxseeds, And Chia Seeds Are Rich In Healthy Fats, Omega-3 Fatty Acids, And Various

Nutrients. They Can Contribute To Heart Health And Provide Satiety.

Yogurt:

• Greek Yogurt And Other Probiotic-Rich Options Support Gut Health. Probiotics May Help With Digestive Issues And Contribute To Overall Well-Being.

Flaxseeds:

• These Seeds Are A Good Source Of Lignans, A Type Of Phytoestrogen. They Also Provide Omega-3 Fatty Acids, Fiber, And May Contribute To Hormonal Balance.

Berries:

• Blueberries, Strawberries, And Raspberries Are Rich In Antioxidants, Vitamins, And Fiber. They Can Contribute To Heart Health And Help Manage Oxidative Stress.

Avocado:

• Avocados Are A Source Of Healthy Monounsaturated Fats, Which Can Support Heart Health And Provide Satiety.

Whole Eggs:

• Eggs Are A Good Source Of Protein, Vitamins, And Minerals. Including Eggs In Your Diet Can Contribute To Overall Nutrient Intake.

Herbs and Spices:

• Incorporate Herbs And Spices Like Turmeric, Ginger, And Cinnamon Into Your Meals. They Not Only Add Flavor But Also Have Anti-Inflammatory Properties.

Water and Herbal Teas:

• Staying Well-Hydrated Is Essential. Water, Herbal Teas, And Infusions Can Help Support Hydration And Contribute To Overall Health.

Remember That Individual Dietary Needs May Vary, And It's Essential To Create A Meal Plan That Suits Your Preferences, Health Status, And Lifestyle. Consulting With A Healthcare Professional Or A

Registered Dietitian Can Provide Personalized Guidance Tailored To Your Specific Needs During Menopause.

Foods to Limit or Avoid

During Menopause, Specific Food Selections Can Aid In Symptom Management And Promote Overall Well-Being. Here Are Several Meals That Should Be Restricted Or Avoided During Menopause:

• Highly Processed Foods, Which Contain Added Sugars, Refined Carbs, And Processed Snacks, Can Lead To Weight Gain And Disturb Blood Sugar Levels. Choose Whole, Unprocessed Meals Instead.

• Consuming An Excessive Amount Of Caffeine Can Worsen Hot Flashes And Disrupt Sleep Patterns. Restrict The Consumption Of Coffee, Tea, And Energy Drinks, Particularly During The Nighttime Hours.

• Excessive Alcohol Drinking Can Disturb Sleep Patterns, Contribute To Weight Gain, And Elevate The Risk Of Osteoporosis. Restrict The Consumption Of Alcohol And Adhere To The Specified Restrictions.

• **Sugary Beverages:** Sugar-Sweetened Beverages Have The Potential To Cause Weight Gain And Have A Detrimental Effect On Metabolic Health. Opt For Water,

Herbal Teas, Or Infused Water As Alternatives.

• Spicy Meals Have The Potential To Provoke Or Intensify Hot Flashes In Certain Women. Observe Your Body's Reaction To Spicy Foods And Contemplate Limiting Consumption If They Cause Any Discomfort.

• Foods With A High Sodium Content: Consuming An Excessive Amount Of Salt Can Lead To Bloating And Could Raise The Likelihood Of Developing High Blood Pressure. Restrict The Intake Of High-Sodium Snacks, Processed Food Products, And Meals From Restaurants And Fast-Food Establishments.

• Consuming Foods That Are High In Fat And Fried Can Lead To Weight Gain And Have A Detrimental Effect On Cardiovascular Health. Opt For More Nutritious Cooking Techniques Like Baking, Grilling, Or Steaming.

• Red And Processed Meats May Include Significant Amounts Of Saturated Fats And Sodium, Which Can Have A Negative Effect On Cardiovascular Health. Choose Low-Fat Protein Options Such As Poultry, Fish, Tofu, And Lentils.

• Dairy Products That Have Been Supplemented With Sugars: O Certain Varieties Of Flavored Yogurts And Sweetened Dairy Products May Contain Additional Sugars. Select

Unadorned, Unsweetened Alternatives And Enhance Them With Your Preferred Fruits Or Nuts To Enhance The Taste.

• Consuming An Excessive Amount Of Dairy Products, Although They Are A Rich Source Of Calcium, May Not Be Necessary And Can Lead To An Increase In Calorie Intake. Select A Range Of Calcium-Rich Food And Contemplate Incorporating Fortified Plant-Based Milk Substitutes.

• **Overconsumption Of Soy Products:** Although Consuming Soy Products In Moderation Is Typically Safe And May Have Health Advantages, Excessive Intake Can Result In An Overconsumption Of Specific

Components. Adopt A Moderate And Well-Rounded Approach To Consuming Soy.

• **White Bread And Refined Grains:** Foods That Are Manufactured With Refined Grains Do Not Have The Fiber And Minerals That Are Present In Whole Grains. Select Whole Grains Such As Brown Rice, Quinoa, And Whole Wheat For Enhanced Nutritional Benefits.

• Certain Artificial Sweeteners May Induce Gastrointestinal Discomfort In Certain Persons. Observe Your Body's Reactions And Select Other Options If Necessary.

- **Fast Food And Takeaway:** Fast Food And Takeaway Meals Frequently Contain Excessive Amounts Of Harmful Fats, Sodium, And Calories. By Cooking Meals At Home With Fresh Ingredients, Individuals Have The Ability To Exert Greater Control Over The Nutritional Composition Of Their Food.

It Is Crucial To Acknowledge That People May Have Varied Reactions To Food, And It Is Recommended To Be Mindful Of How Your Body Responds To Various Dietary Options. Furthermore, Seeking Advice From A Healthcare Expert Or Certified Dietitian Can Offer Tailored Recommendations Based On Your

Own Health Requirements And Personal Preferences Throughout Menopause.

CHAPTER FOUR
Superfoods for Menopause

While The Term "Superfood" Is Not A Scientific Classification, It Is Commonly Used To Describe Nutrient-Dense Foods That Offer A Variety Of Health Benefits. During Menopause, Including Range Of Nutrient-Rich Foods In Your Diet Can Be Particularly Beneficial. Here Are Some Foods Often Considered As "Superfoods" That Can Be Beneficial During Menopause:

• **Fatty Fish (Salmon, Mackerel, Sardines):** Rich In Omega-3 Fatty Acids, These Fish Can Support Heart Health, Reduce Inflammation, And Potentially Help Manage Mood Swings And Joint Pain.

• **Flaxseeds:** High In Lignans, Fiber, And Omega-3 Fatty Acids, Flaxseeds May Help Alleviate Menopausal Symptoms, Such As Hot Flashes And Mood Swings.

• **Soy Products (Tofu, Edamame, Soy Milk):** Soy Contains Phytoestrogens, Which Have Mild Estrogenic Effects. Incorporating Soy Into The Diet May Help Manage Certain Menopausal Symptoms.

• **Berries (Blueberries, Strawberries, Raspberries):** Berries Are Rich In Antioxidants, Vitamins, And Fiber, Supporting Heart Health And Helping Manage Oxidative Stress.

• **Leafy Greens (Spinach, Kale, Swiss Chard):** Packed With Calcium, Magnesium, Vitamin K, And Other Nutrients, Leafy Greens Are Essential For Bone Health During Menopause.

• **Greek Yogurt:** A Good Source Of Calcium And Probiotics, Greek Yogurt Supports Bone Health And Contributes To Gut Health.

• **Nuts and Seeds (Almonds, Walnuts, Chia Seeds):** Provide Healthy Fats, Protein, And Essential Nutrients. Nuts And Seeds Can Be Beneficial For Heart Health And Satiety.

- **Broccoli and Cruciferous Vegetables:** Contain Compounds That May Support Detoxification And Promote Overall Health. They Also Provide Fiber, Vitamins, And Minerals.

- **Avocado:** Rich In Monounsaturated Fats, Avocados Can Contribute To Heart Health And Provide A Feeling Of Satiety.

- **Whole Grains (Quinoa, Brown Rice, Oats):** Provide Complex Carbohydrates, Fiber, And Essential Nutrients. Whole Grains Support Sustained Energy Levels And Digestive Health.

• **Turmeric:** Contains Curcumin, Which Has Anti-Inflammatory Properties. Turmeric May Help Manage Inflammation And Joint Pain.

• **Green Tea:** A Low-Calorie Beverage Rich In Antioxidants, Green Tea May Contribute To Weight Management And Reduce The Frequency Of Hot Flashes.

• **Pumpkin Seeds:** High In Magnesium, Zinc, and Omega-3 Fatty Acids, Pumpkin Seeds Can Support Bone Health And Potentially Alleviate Certain Symptoms.

• **Cottage Cheese:** A Good Source Of Protein And Calcium, Cottage Cheese Supports Muscle Health And Bone Health.

• **Tomatoes:** Contain Lycopene, An Antioxidant That May Contribute To Heart Health. Cooking Tomatoes Enhances The Absorption Of Lycopene.

It Is Crucial To Bear In Mind That Although These Foods Provide Different Health Advantages, A Comprehensive And Varied Diet Is Essential. Furthermore, It Is Prudent To Seek Guidance From Healthcare Specialists Or Qualified Dietitians To Obtain Specific Recommendations Tailored To Individual Health

Requirements And Preferences During Menopause, As Individual Reactions To Food Can Differ.

Weight Management during Menopause

Weight Management During Menopause Can Be Difficult Because Of Hormonal Fluctuations, Alterations In Metabolism, And Changes In Lifestyle. Nevertheless, Embracing Wholesome Behaviors Can Aid In Sustaining A Desirable Weight And Fostering General Wellness. Below Are Few Techniques For Effectively Maintaining Weight During Menopause:

• **Balanced Diet:** Focus On A Well-Balanced Diet That Includes A Variety Of Nutrient-Dense Foods. Include Plenty Of Fruits, Vegetables, Whole Grains, Lean Proteins, And Healthy Fats. Aim For Portion Control To Manage Calorie Intake.

• **Lean Protein:** Prioritize Lean Protein Sources Such As Poultry, Fish, Tofu, Legumes, And Nuts. Protein Helps Maintain Muscle Mass, Support Metabolism, And Provides A Feeling Of Fullness.

• **Whole Grains:** Choose Whole Grains Over Refined Grains For Better Fiber Content And Sustained Energy. Options Like Quinoa, Brown Rice, Oats, And Whole Wheat Are Good Choices.

• **Healthy Fats:** Include Sources Of Healthy Fats In Your Diet, Such As Avocados, Nuts, Seeds, And Olive Oil. These Fats Contribute To Satiety And Provide Essential Nutrients.

• **Portion Control:** Be Mindful Of Portion Sizes To Avoid Overeating. Pay Attention To Hunger And Fullness Cues And Avoid Eating In Front Of Screens To Promote Mindful Eating.

• **Stay Hydrated:** Drink Plenty Of Water Throughout The Day. Sometimes, The Body Can Confuse Thirst With Hunger. Staying Hydrated Can Help Manage Appetite And Support Overall Health.

- **Regular Physical Activity:** Incorporate Regular Exercise Into Your Routine. Both Cardiovascular Exercises (E.G., Brisk Walking, Cycling) And Strength Training Can Help Manage Weight, Boost Metabolism, And Support Overall Well-Being.

- **Resistance Training:** Include Resistance Training Or Strength-Building Exercises To Maintain And Build Muscle Mass. Muscle Burns More Calories At Rest Than Fat, Contributing To A Healthy Metabolism.

- **Manage Stress:** Chronic Stress Can Contribute To Weight Gain. Practice Stress Management Techniques Such As Meditation, Yoga, Deep Breathing, Or Hobbies To Reduce Stress Levels.

- **Adequate Sleep:** Lack Of Sleep Can Disrupt Hormones That Regulate Hunger And Satiety. Aim For 7-9 Hours Of Quality Sleep Per Night To Support Weight Management.

- **Limit Processed Foods And Added Sugars:** Processed Foods And Added Sugars Can Contribute To Excess Calorie Intake. Limit The Consumption Of Sugary Snacks, Sodas, And Highly Processed Foods.

- **Regular Health Check-Ups:** Schedule Regular Check-Ups With Your Healthcare Provider To Monitor Overall Health, Discuss Weight Management Strategies, And Address Any Specific Concerns Related To Menopause.

• **Hormone Replacement Therapy (HRT) Consideration:** In Some Cases, Hormone Replacement Therapy (HRT) May Be Considered Under The Guidance Of Healthcare Professionals. HRT Can Help Manage Certain Menopausal Symptoms And Potentially Contribute To Weight Management.

When Dealing With Weight Management During Menopause, It Is Crucial To Adopt A Comprehensive Approach That Emphasizes Total Well-Being Rather Than Just Fixating On One's Weight. Seeking Advice From Healthcare Professionals, Such As A Certified Dietitian Or Fitness Expert, Can Offer Customized Assistance That

Is   Specifically   Designed   To   Meet
Individual Needs And Preferences.

CHAPTER FIVE
Managing Individual Menopausal Symptoms with Dietary Interventions

Nutrition Can Have An Impact On Managing Particular Symptoms Associated With Menopause. Although Dietary Adjustments May Not Completely Eradicate Symptoms, They Can Effectively Mitigate And Relieve Specific Discomforts. Below Are Dietary Approaches That Target Certain Symptoms Experienced During Menopause:

Hot Flashes and Night Sweats:

• **Avoid Trigger Foods:** Some Women Find That Certain Foods And Drinks, Such As Spicy Foods, Caffeine, And

Alcohol, Can Trigger Hot Flashes. Identifying And Limiting These Triggers May Help Reduce The Frequency And Intensity Of Hot Flashes.

• **Include Phytoestrogens**: Foods Rich In Phytoestrogens, Like Soy Products (Tofu, Edamame), Flaxseeds, And Whole Grains, May Have Mild Estrogenic Effects And Could Help Alleviate Hot Flashes.

Vaginal Dryness:

• **Stay Hydrated:** Drinking Enough Water Helps Maintain Overall Hydration, Including Vaginal Moisture.

• **Omega-3 Fatty Acids:** Include Foods Rich In Omega-3 Fatty Acids, Such As

Fatty Fish, Flaxseeds, And Chia Seeds, Which May Support Skin And Mucosal Health.

Mood Swings and Irritability:

• **Balanced Diet:** A Balanced Diet With Adequate Nutrients Supports Mood Regulation. Include Complex Carbohydrates, Lean Proteins, And Healthy Fats.

• **B Vitamins:** Foods Rich In B Vitamins (Whole Grains, Legumes, Nuts, Seeds, Leafy Greens) Are Essential For Neurotransmitter Function And May Help Stabilize Mood.

Sleep Disturbances:

• **Limit Caffeine:** Reduce Or Avoid Caffeine, Especially In The Afternoon And Evening, To Improve Sleep Quality.

• **Melatonin-Rich Foods:** Include Foods With Melatonin, Such As Cherries, Tomatoes, And Grapes, Which May Help Regulate Sleep.

Joint Pain and Muscle Aches:

• **Omega-3 Fatty Acids:** Incorporate Foods Rich In Omega-3 Fatty Acids To Reduce Inflammation And Support Joint Health.

• **Calcium And Vitamin D:** Ensure An Adequate Intake Of Calcium And

Vitamin D For Bone Health, Which Can Contribute To Overall Joint Health.

Weight Gain:

• **Balanced Diet And Portion Control:** Focus On A Balanced Diet With Appropriate Portion Sizes To Manage Calorie Intake.

• **Regular Exercise:** Include Both Cardiovascular And Strength Training Exercises To Support Metabolism And Maintain Muscle Mass.

Cognitive Function (Brain Fog):

• Omega-3 Fatty Acids: Foods Rich in Omega-3 Fatty Acids Can Support Brain Health and Cognitive Function.

- **Antioxidant-Rich Foods:** Include Colorful Fruits And Vegetables With Antioxidants To Protect Against Oxidative Stress.

Urinary Changes:

- **Fluid Balance:** Maintain Proper Hydration To Support Urinary Health.

- **Kegel Exercises:** In Addition To Diet, Pelvic Floor Exercises (Kegels) Can Help With Urinary Incontinence.

Bone Health (Osteoporosis Prevention):

- **Calcium And Vitamin D:** Ensure Adequate Intake Of Calcium And Vitamin D Through Dairy Products, Fortified Plant-Based Milk, Leafy Greens, And Exposure To Sunlight.

• **Vitamin K:** Include Foods Rich In Vitamin K, Such As Leafy Greens And Broccoli, To Support Bone Health.

It's Important To Note That Individual Responses To Dietary Changes Vary. Consulting With Healthcare Professionals Or A Registered Dietitian Can Provide Personalized Guidance Tailored To Specific Symptoms, Health Conditions, And Dietary Preferences During Menopause.

Types of Exercise for Menopausal Women

Physical Activity Is Essential For Maintaining Good Health And A Sense Of Well-Being, And It Can Have Particularly Positive Effects During The Menopausal Period. Participating

In A Diverse Range Of Activities, Such As Aerobic, Strength Training, Flexibility, And Balance Exercises, Can Effectively Aid In Weight Management, Promote Bone Health, Ease Mood Swings, And Enhance Sleep Quality. Below Are Many Exercises That Are Appropriate For Ladies Experiencing Menopause:

1. Cardiovascular Exercise:

- **Walking:** A Low-Impact Activity That Is Easy To Incorporate Into Daily Life.
- Cycling: Stationary or Outdoor Cycling Provides a Good Cardiovascular Workout.

- **Swimming:** A Low-Impact Exercise That Is Gentle On The Joints.

- **Dancing:** Fun And Effective For Cardiovascular Health.

- **Aerobic Classes:** Joining Group Classes Can Provide Motivation And Variety.

Strength Training:

- **Weightlifting:** Incorporate Resistance Training Using Dumbbells, Resistance Bands, Or Weight Machines To Build And Maintain Muscle Mass.

- **Bodyweight Exercises:** Include Squats, Lunges, Push-Ups, And Planks For Strength Training Without Equipment.

- **Yoga And Pilates:** While Emphasizing Flexibility And Balance, These Exercises Also Engage Muscles To Improve Strength.

Flexibility and Stretching:

- **Yoga:** Combines Flexibility, Strength, and Relaxation.
- **Pilates:** Focuses On Core Strength, Flexibility, And Overall Body Awareness.
- **Tai Chi:** A Slow And Controlled Form Of Exercise That Enhances Flexibility And Balance.
- **Static Stretching:** Include Stretches For Major Muscle Groups After Your Workout To Improve Flexibility.

Balance Exercises:

- **Tai Chi**: Besides Flexibility, Tai Chi Also Enhances Balance And Coordination.

- **Single-Leg Stands:** Stand On One Leg For Short Durations To Improve Balance.

- **Balance Exercises on Unstable Surfaces:** Use Stability Balls Or Balance Pads To Challenge And Improve Stability.

Core Exercises:

- **Pilates:** Many Pilates Exercises Focus On The Core.

- **Planks**: Effective For Engaging The Core Muscles.

- **Abdominal Exercises:** Include Exercises Like Crunches And Twists To Strengthen The Abdominal Muscles.

Mind-Body Exercises:

Yoga and Pilates: Both Incorporate Mindfulness And Breathing Techniques.

Meditation: Can Help Manage Stress And Improve Overall Well-Being.

High-Intensity Interval Training (HIIT):

• **Short Bursts Of Intense Exercise:** Alternating Between Intense Bursts Of Activity And Rest Periods Can Be Time-Efficient And Effective For Cardiovascular Health.

Outdoor Activities:

- **Hiking:** A Great Way To Combine Cardiovascular Exercise With Nature.

- **Gardening:** Engaging In Gardening Activities Can Provide A Low-Impact Workout.

Before Starting Any New Exercise Program, It's Advisable For Menopausal Women To Consult With Healthcare Professionals, Especially If There Are Existing Health Conditions. A Personalized Exercise Plan That Takes Into Account Individual Fitness Levels, Preferences, And Health Considerations Is Important For Long-Term Adherence And Success. Additionally, Listening To The Body,

Staying Hydrated, And Incorporating A Mix Of Activities For Variety Can Contribute To A Well-Rounded Exercise Routine During Menopause.

Supplements for Menopause

While It's Generally Prefer able To Obtain Nutrients From A Well-Balanced Diet, Some Women May Benefit From Supplements During Menopause To Address Specific Nutritional Needs. It's Important To Consult With A Healthcare Professional Before Adding Any Supplements To Your Routine, As Individual Needs Can Vary. Here Are Some Supplements That Are Commonly Considered For Menopausal Women:

Calcium and Vitamin D:

• **Importance:** Essential For Bone Health, Especially As Estrogen Levels Decline During Menopause.

• **Sources:** Dairy Products, Fortified Plant-Based Milk, Leafy Greens, And Exposure To Sunlight.

• **Supplementation:** If Dietary Intake Is Insufficient, Calcium And Vitamin D Supplements May Be Recommended.

Omega-3 Fatty Acids:

• **Importance:** Support Cardiovascular Health, Reduce Inflammation, And May Help Manage Mood Swings.

- **Sources:** Fatty Fish (Salmon, Mackerel, Sardines), Flaxseeds, Chia Seeds, Walnuts.

- **Supplementation:** Fish Oil Or Algae-Based Omega-3 Supplements Can Be Considered.

Magnesium:

- **Importance:** Supports Bone Health, Muscle Function, And May Help With Sleep And Mood Regulation.

- **Sources:** Nuts, Seeds, Whole Grains, Leafy Green Vegetables.

- **Supplementation:** Magnesium Supplements May Be Considered If Dietary Intake Is Insufficient.

Vitamin K:

- **Importance:** Important For Bone Health And Blood Clotting.

- **Sources:** Leafy Green Vegetables (Kale, Spinach, Broccoli), Brussels Sprouts.

- **Supplementation:** If Dietary Intake Is Low, Vitamin K Supplements Can Be Considered.

Vitamin B Complex:

- **Importance:** B Vitamins, Including B6, B12, and Folate, Support Energy Metabolism and Nervous System Function.

• **Sources:** Whole Grains, Lean Meats, Fish, Poultry, Dairy Products, Legumes.

• **Supplementation**: In Some Cases, B-Complex Supplements May Be Recommended, Especially For Those With Dietary Restrictions.

Vitamin C:

• **Importance:** An Antioxidant That Supports The Immune System And Helps Absorb Iron.

• **Sources:** Citrus Fruits, Strawberries, Bell Peppers, Broccoli.

• **Supplementation:** Generally Unnecessary If A Well-Balanced Diet Is Maintained.

Soy is flavones Or Phytoestrogens:

• **Importance:** May Help Alleviate Certain Menopausal Symptoms Due To Their Mild Estrogenic Effects.

• **Sources:** Soy Products (Tofu, Edamame), Flaxseeds, Whole Grains.

• **Supplementation:** Soy Isoflavone Supplements Can Be Considered, But It's Advisable To Get These Compounds From Food Sources.

Black Cohosh:

• **Importance:** Traditionally Used To Manage Hot Flashes And Other Menopausal Symptoms.

• **Sources:** Extracted From The Root Of The Black Cohosh Plant.

- **Supplementation:** Black Cohosh Supplements Are Available, But Their Efficacy Varies, And Consultation With A Healthcare Professional Is Recommended.

Probiotics:

- **Importance:** Support Gut Health And May Contribute To Overall Well-Being, Including Vaginal Health.

- **Sources:** Yogurt, Kefir, Fermented Foods.

- **Supplementation:** Probiotic Supplements Can Be Considered, Especially For Those Who May Not Consume Fermented Foods Regularly.

Always Consult With A Healthcare Professional Before Starting Any New

Supplement Regimen, As Excessive Intake Of Certain Nutrients Can Have Adverse Effects. Additionally, Individual Needs And Potential Interactions With Medications Should Be Taken Into Consideration. A Personalized Approach, Including Regular Health Check-Ups And Discussions With A Healthcare Provider, Is Crucial During Menopause.

CHAPTER SIX
Meal Planning and Recipes

Meal Planning During Menopause Entails Designing Meals That Are Both Well-Balanced And Nutrient-Dense, With The Aim Of Addressing Specific Nutritional Requirements And Effectively Managing Symptoms Commonly Associated With This Particular Phase Of Life. Below Is A Sample Meal Plan Accompanied With Corresponding Recipes:

Sample Meal Plan:

Breakfast:

Quinoa Breakfast Bowl:

- Cooked Quinoa
- Greek Yogurt

- Fresh Berries (Blueberries, Strawberries)
- Chopped Nuts (Almonds, Walnuts)
- Drizzle Of Honey

Mid-Morning Snack:

Green Smoothie:

- Spinach
- Banana
- Greek Yogurt
- Chia Seeds
- Almond Milk

Lunch:

Salmon and Avocado Salad:

- Grilled Salmon Fillet

- Mixed Greens (Spinach, Arugula, Kale)
- Cherry Tomatoes
- Cucumber Slices
- Avocado
- Olive Oil And Lemon Dressing

Afternoon Snack:

Greek Yogurt Parfait:

- Greek Yogurt
- Granola
- Mixed Berries
- Drizzle Of Maple Syrup

Dinner:

Vegetarian Stir-Fry:

- Tofu or Tempeh

- Mixed Vegetables (Broccoli, Bell Peppers, Snap Peas)
- Brown Rice Or Quinoa
- Soy Sauce And Ginger Sauce

Evening Snack:

• Handful of Almonds or Walnuts

Recipes:

Quinoa Breakfast Bowl:

- Cook Quinoa According To Package Instructions.
- In A Bowl, Layer Cooked Quinoa, Greek Yogurt, Fresh Berries, And Chopped Nuts.
- Drizzle With Honey for Sweetness.

Green Smoothie:

• Blend Together Spinach, Banana, Greek Yogurt, Chia Seeds, And Almond Milk Until Smooth.

Salmon and Avocado Salad:

- Grill Salmon Fillet And Let It Cool.
- In A Large Bowl, Combine Mixed Greens, Cherry Tomatoes, Cucumber Slices, And Diced Avocado.
- Top With Grilled Salmon.
- Drizzle With Olive Oil And Lemon Dressing.

Greek Yogurt Parfait:

- In A Glass or Bowl, Layer Greek Yogurt with Granola And Mixed Berries.
- Drizzle With A Touch Of Maple Syrup For Sweetness.

Vegetarian Stir-Fry:

- Cut Tofu or Tempeh into Cubes.
- Stir-Fry Mixed Vegetables And Tofu/Tempeh In A Pan With Soy Sauce And Ginger Sauce.
- Serve Over Brown Rice Or Quinoa.

These Dishes Offer A Harmonious Combination Of Protein, Nutritious Fats, And Intricate Carbs, As Well As A Diverse Range Of Vitamins And

Minerals. Modify The Amount Of Food Served According To The Specific Requirements And Desires Of Each Person.

Ensure Proper Hydration By Consuming Ample Amounts Of Water Throughout The Day. Furthermore, It Is Advisable To Include Herbs And Spices Into Your Cooking To Enhance The Taste And Potentially Gain Health Advantages. Seeking Guidance From A Healthcare Expert Or A Qualified Dietitian Can Assist In Developing A Customized Meal Plan Tailored To Individual Health Requirements And Preferences Throughout The Menopausal Period.

Techniques for Managing Stress

Effectively Managing Stress Is Imperative During Menopause, Since The Hormonal Fluctuations And Accompanying Symptoms Can Significantly Contribute To Elevated Stress Levels. Integrating Stress Management Practices Into Your Daily Schedule Can Enhance Your Overall State Of Well-Being. Below Are Few Efficacious Stress Mitigation Strategies Specifically Tailored For Menopausal Women:

- **Engage In Deep Breathing Exercises:** Employ Deep Breathing Techniques To Soothe The Nervous System. Breathe In Deeply Through Your Nostrils, Retain The Breath For A

Brief Period, And Then Release It Slowly Via Your Oral Cavity. Reiterate Many Times.

• Practice Mindfulness Meditation To Cultivate Conscious Awareness Of The Present Moment. Direct Your Attention On Your Breath, The Sensations Within Your Body, Or A Soothing Mantra.

• Yoga Is A Practice That Involves The Integration Of Physical Postures, Breath Control, And Meditation. Consistent Practice Can Strengthen Flexibility, Alleviate Tension, And Improve General Well-Being.

• Progressive Muscle Relaxation (PMR) Is A Technique That Involves

Deliberately Tensing And Subsequently Relaxing Various Muscle Groups In Order To Alleviate Physical Tension. This Approach Induces A State Of Calm In The Entire Body.

• **Guided Imagery:** Envision A Serene And Tranquil Setting. This Can Aid In Redirecting Your Attention From Worries And Fostering A Feeling Of Serenity.

• **Consistent Physical Activity:** Participate In Frequent Exercise, Such As Walking, Running, Swimming, Or Dancing. Physical Activity Stimulates The Release Of Endorphins, Which Are Naturally Occurring Substances That Elevate Mood.

- **Journaling:** Document Your Ideas And Emotions In A Personal Journal. This Activity Can Serve As A Means Of Expressing Oneself And Aid In Recognizing Recurring Patterns Or Factors That Cause Stress.

- **Social Support:** Establish Connections With Friends, Family, Or Support Groups. Engaging In The Act Of Expressing Your Emotions And Recounting Your Personal Experiences To Others Can Offer Valuable Emotional Assistance And A Broader Outlook.

- **Efficient Time Management:** Arrange And Rank Tasks In Order To Properly Manage Your Time. Divide

Huge Jobs Into Smaller, More Feasible Segments.

• **Aromatherapy:** Employ Soothing Fragrances like Lavender, Chamomile, Or Bergamot. Aromatherapy Can Be Employed For Relaxation, Utilizing Essential Oils Or Scented Candles.

• **Utilize Laughing Therapy:** Engage In Activities Such As Watching A Humorous Film, Attending A Comedy Concert, Or Socializing With Those Who Have The Ability To Induce Laughter. Laughter Possesses The Inherent Ability To Alleviate Stress.

• **Minimize Stimulants:** Decrease The Consumption Of Stimulants Like

Caffeine And Nicotine, As These Might Exacerbate Stress Levels.

• Optimize The Quality Of Your Sleep By Prioritizing Sleep Hygiene To Guarantee A Restorative And Undisturbed Night's Rest. Adhere To A Regular Sleep Schedule And Establish A Soothing Nighttime Routine.

• **Optimal Nutrition:** Consume A Diet That Is Well-Rounded, Emphasizing Foods That Are Rich In Nutrients. Adequate Nutrition Has The Potential To Have A Beneficial Effect On Both The Physical And Mental State Of An Individual.

• If Stress Becomes Unmanageable, It Is Advisable To Seek Assistance From

A Mental Health Expert. Therapists Or Counselors Can Offer Techniques For Managing Stress And Provide Assistance In Dealing With Emotions.

It Is Crucial To Investigate Various Stress Management Strategies In Order To Determine The Most Effective Approach For Oneself. Integrating Various Tactics Into Your Daily Routine Can Enhance Your Overall Approach To Managing Stress During Menopause.

Conclusion

Ultimately, Menopause Is An Inherent Phase In A Woman's Existence That Entails Hormonal Alterations And A Range Of Physical And Mental Symptoms. Although This Stage May Present Difficulties, Women Can Make It Easier And More Comfortable By Embracing A Comprehensive Approach That Encompasses Appropriate Nutrition, Consistent Physical Activity, Stress Management Strategies, And, If Needed, The Use Of Supplements.

• An Optimally Balanced Diet Abundant In Essential Minerals Such As Calcium, Omega-3 Fatty Acids, And Phytoestrogens Can Promote Overall

Well-Being And Ease Particular Symptoms Associated With Menopause. Participating In A Diverse Range Of Exercises, Such As Aerobic, Strength Training, Flexibility, And Balancing Exercises, Can Effectively Control Weight, Promote Bone Health, And Enhance Mood And Sleep Quality.

• Stress Management Practices, Including Deep Breathing, Mindfulness Meditation, Yoga, And Social Support, Are Crucial For Dealing With The Emotional And Psychological Components Of Menopause. Furthermore, It Is Imperative To Uphold An Optimistic Outlook, Seek Assistance From Experts When Necessary, And Maintain Regular

Communication With Healthcare Specialists For Direction And Assistance In Properly Managing Menopause.

By Adopting A Proactive Stance Towards Menopause And Embracing Healthy Living Practices, Women Can Successfully Navigate This Transitional Phase With Strength, Energy, And A Feeling Of Empowerment. It Is Crucial To Bear In Mind That Each Woman's Encounter With Menopause Is Distinct, Thus Discovering Tailored Approaches That Are Most Effective For You Is Essential For Maximizing Your Overall Well-Being During This Phase Of Life.

THE END